Aromatherapy

A Guide for Beginners

I0417539

Reap the Benefits of Using Essential Oils In Your Life

RON KNESS

ISBN-13: 978-1540666161

ISBN-10: 1540666166

Contents

Disclaimer

This publication is for informational purposes only and is not intended as medical advice. Medical advice should always be obtained from a qualified medical professional for any health conditions or symptoms associated with them. Every possible effort has been made in preparing and researching this material. We make no warranties with respect to the accuracy, applicability of its contents or any omissions.

Essential oils are highly concentrated and not all of them are safe for internal use so be sure to check the safety of any oil before digesting. If you are pregnant, some oils can cause contractions, always ask your doctor before use.

Topical application requires dilution with a carrier oil as some oils can cause skin irritation when used in their original high concentration form.

Every possible effort has been made in preparing and researching this material. We make no warranties with respect to the accuracy, applicability of its contents or any omissions.

See your healthcare professional before starting any diet or exercise program!

Introduction

Aromatherapy is the practice of using essential oils from plants for the purpose of healing. The Chinese have been using this method of relaxation and healing for centuries. There are numerous ways you can use essential oils. Some of the most popular approaches are inhalation, massaging essential oils into the skin, and mixing them with face creams and body lotions.

By applying essential oils properly, you'll experience a great

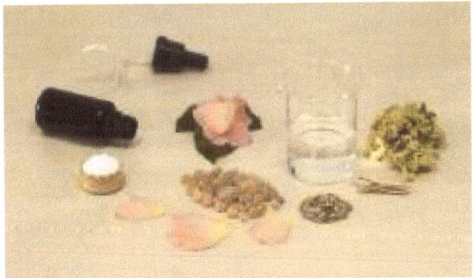

alternative treatment for stress, fatigue, insomnia and many other health problems. Aromatherapy is also well known for improving mood and providing wonderful healing scents that promote general wellness and wellbeing.

What Are Essential Oils?

Essential oils are oils extracted from various plants and botanicals. They are oils that are therapeutic grade and hold medicinal value, highly concentrated and pure.

Various processes are used to extract these oils, which include:

- Steam Distillation

- Expression

- Solvent Extraction

- Absolute Oil Extraction

- Resin Tapping

- Cold Pressing

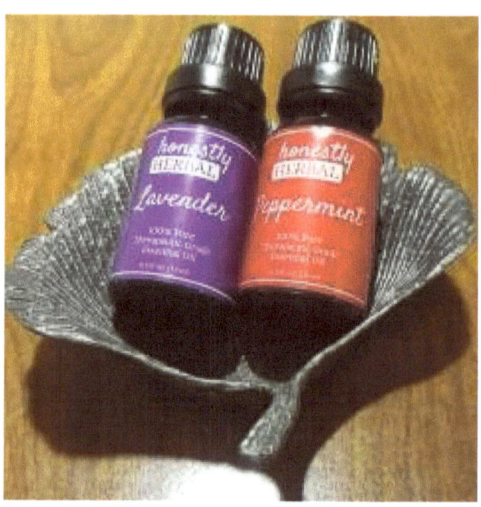

Each different oil has its own therapeutic value; each extract has its own yield of active ingredients, which determines what it is going to be used for and/or its healing properties.

For example, certain essential oils are used to enhance relaxation and reduce stress; others can help alleviate nausea and boost energy. There are even oils that can be used as antiseptics and in household cleaners.

Essential oils have been used throughout history as an alternative medicine for various conditions, and general wellness and wellbeing.

While traditional, evidence-based medicine has experienced a decline in the use of essential oils, there are still many people who prefer to use essential oils as a natural alternative, even if it is just to relax and create a certain mood.

There are many different medicinal uses for essential oils, but they are also often used to replace commercial chemical-laden cleaners and beauty products for homemade skin and hair care, and household use.

Aromatherapy History

Although aromatherapy seems like it's becoming more popular with each passing year, the use of essential oils for therapeutic purposes dates back to 6,000 years ago. The ancient Romans, Indians, Chinese, Greeks, and Egyptians all used them for hygienic, therapeutic, ritualistic, and spiritual purposes.

More than 2,500 years ago, Hippocrates noted that aromatic baths had a significant impact on the overall well-being of an individual. During the early 19th century, essential oils started being present in

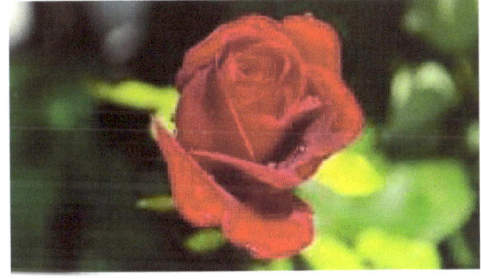

western medicine practices, while later on in the century, both German and French medical professors started using them to fight infected wounds.

However, it was not until 1928 that the actual science of aromatherapy was born. The discovery was made by a French chemist named René-Maurice Gattefossé when there was an explosion in his laboratory, and he had suffered a burn on his hand. In an attempt to heal it quickly, he applied lavender oil on his skin, and was pleasantly surprised to find out that it worked.

Afterwards, Gattefossé started reading about how certain essential oils were used to treat wounds, burns, gangrene, and skin infections during World War I.

By the 1950s, a lot beauticians, doctors, and massage therapists started recommending aromatherapy. However, it didn't become that popular until the 1980s.

Nowadays, the use of therapeutic grade essential oils is commonplace. In addition, there are numerous candles, beauty products, and lotions sold as 'aromatherapy' in a number of stores. Note that these products won't actually help you the way therapeutic grade essential oils will, because they mostly contain synthetic fragrances.

Uses for Essential Oils

The great thing about essential oils is they can be used in a number of different ways:

Health and Wellness: Of course, there are many more ways you will benefit from using essential oils other than simply enjoying their smell. If you want to boost your energy, get better sleep, or overcome a bad mood, then aromatherapy is always a good idea.

Relaxation: If you often suffer from headaches or experience high levels of stress, then you really need to start using essential oils as soon as possible. They will not only help keep you relaxed, but they will also help you get a higher quality of sleep.

To Enhance Mood: Sometimes it's really hard to get out of a bad mood. However, the good news is that essential oils can help you when it comes to enhancing your mood. There are oils that can inspire feelings of romance, relaxation, calm, peace, energy, happiness and to release anger and frustration.

Home and Household: One of the most popular uses for aromatherapy is to clean and freshen the air in a household. Even if you live in an area that is surrounded by nature and constantly keep your windows open, you can still benefit from using essential oils to create a more pleasant aura in your home. Oils can also be used for various household needs, such as in homemade cleaners or in laundry.

Home Remedies: There are various oils that can be used as home remedies for minor conditions.

Beauty, Homemade Skin Care and Hygiene Products:
Many essential oils are used in creams, shampoos, and
many different personal hygiene products. There are many
recipes for all types of beauty purposes, and many take
advantage of these to make homemade products.

They can be used topically to treat a variety of skin and pain
conditions, or used in baths to treat aches and pains as well
as colds and flus.

You can also use essential oils in cleaning products,
cosmetics, aromatherapy, and even to flavor food and
drinks.

Aromatherapy diffusers are used to infuse the air you
breathe with essential oils for both their scent and
therapeutic value.

It is recommended that essential oils always be diluted
before using them on the skin or ingesting them, as they can
cause skin irritation. Olive oil makes a good "carrier oil" for
dilution.

Health Benefits of Aromatherapy

Improved Sleep Quality

Many aromatherapy oils will help decrease stress levels and help you unwind, which will in turn provide you with improved sleep quality. Some of the best sleep-inducing essential oils include vetiver, rose, lavender, ylang-ylang, and chamomile.

Relaxation And Mood

Chamomile and lavender are wonderful scents that help induce the relaxation response in the body to reduce stress and its harmful effects. They are also wonderful mood enhancers that promote feelings of calm and peace. These oils can be enjoyed in an aromatherapy diffuser, in a hot bath or by placing a few drops on your pillow before going to sleep. Chamomile also makes for a relaxing tea before going to bed.

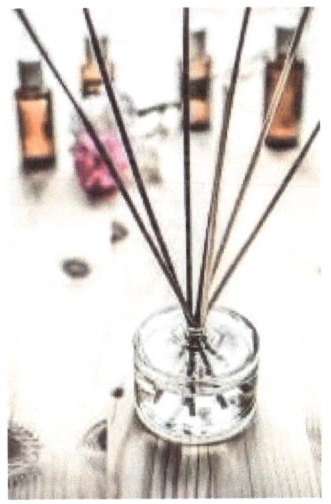

Reduce Stress and Anxiety

Lavender, rose, vetiver, ylang-ylang, bergamot, chamomile, marjoram and frankincense are the best essential oils to reduce nervousness, anxiety and stress. These are calm inspiring scents that are soothing, cheerful, and relaxing.

Reduced Nausea And Improved Digestion

The essential oils known for providing you with these health benefits include lemon, grapefruit, peppermint, ginger, eucalyptus, turmeric, and chamomile. They can help alleviate indigestion, ulcer pain, morning sickness, and nausea.

Improved Skin Health

The best oil to treat skin problems is without doubt tea tree oil. It is noted for its antiseptic, antifungal, and antibacterial properties. Other essential oils that improve skin health are orange, juniper berry, frankincense, clary sage, lemon, and lavender. When spritzed to the skin or scalp, they are able to reduce dandruff, toe fungus, itching, cellulite, and rashes. These oils are also known for improving wound healing.

Energy Boost

Most of us depend on certain stimulants to provide us with

energy throughout the day, such as coffee, or energy drinks. However, these stimulants can have an incredibly bad effect on our body.

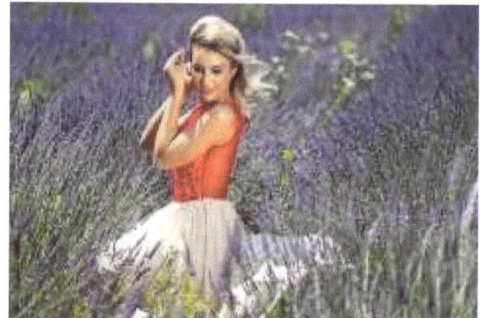

Although some choose to exercise and eat healthy in order to increase their energy levels, it wouldn't hurt if you were to add some aromatherapy into the mix. Essential oils like cinnamon, tea tree, sage, angelica, rosemary, cardamom, and jasmine are known for increasing circulation and raising energy levels.

Improved Memory

As you grow older, you'll be experiencing more and more problems with your memory. Even though you can't fully combat the negative effects of aging, there are certain ways for you to slow down this process. Aromatherapy with sage oil is often used as an alternative treatment for dementia and it is also noted for helping anyone boost his or her memory capacity.

Headaches

We all get headaches from time to time and some suffer from the more intense migraines that can really affect quality of life and ruin a whole day. The most common essential oils used to reduce migraines and headaches are rosemary, eucalyptus, peppermint, and sandalwood. These oils are usually mixed with almond, coconut, jojoba, or avocado oils before being applied to the skin and/or scalp.

Improved Immune System

Most medical professionals agree that prevention is a smart road to good health, which is a great reason to start using aromatherapy. Thanks to the antibacterial and anti-fungal properties of essential oils such as peppermint, lemon, cinnamon, eucalyptus, and oregano, they can help improve your immune system and protect you from numerous illnesses and infections.

Pain Relief

Pain relief is without a doubt one of the most useful health benefits of aromatherapy. The best essential oils for pain relief are eucalyptus, chamomile, clary sage, lavender, rosemary, juniper, and peppermint.

Often, by simply inducing a relaxation response with the use of relaxation promoting essential oils in a diffuser, such as lavender and chamomile, you can help reduce the perception of pain.

These oils can be mixed with carrier oils for use in massage. Another way to help pain is to add a few drops of oil into a warm bath.

What Are the Benefits of the Different Essential Oils?

There are many different flavors of essential oils on the market, each with their own uses and benefits. We discussed some of the more general uses of some, but below is a more in-depth usage of each one. Here are a few of the most popular.

Lavender

It's no wonder that René-Maurice Gattefossé founded the

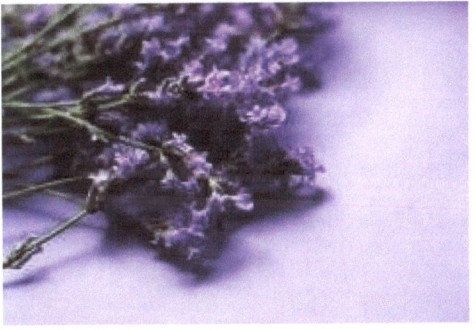

whole science of aromatherapy after identifying the healing effects of this particular essential oil. Lavender is mostly used for reducing stress levels and relaxation. However, it is also known for helping to fight against the flu, migraines, and colds.

In order to get a good night's sleep, you can either add a few drops to an aromatherapy diffuser or straight onto your pillow. If you want to relax before going to bed, add a few drops of lavender oil into your hot or warm bath.

Tea Tree

If you had to choose, just one essential oil from the numerous available, tea tree oil would be a great choice.

Even though lavender is historically important, tea tree is equally popular and important. It is best known for fighting infections and boosting the immune system.

However, it's worth noting that there are numerous other healing properties of tea tree. It heals skin conditions, cuts (avoid using it for serious cuts) and burns, it boosts the immune system, treats cold sores, and muscle aches.

On top of that, it can also treat respiratory conditions. Even though this essential oil isn't toxic, it shouldn't be used around the nose and eyes, or internally. Tea Tree oil can be applied directly to the skin when blended with a carrier oil, added to bathwater, and/or inhaled.

Ylang-Ylang

Ylang-Ylang has a strong scent and is used for reducing stress, and also serves as an aphrodisiac. This essential oil can be blended with carrier oils and used for massages, or added to a diffuser. If you're planning a romantic bath with your significant other, you can also add a few drops into a bath.

Even though it is mostly used for calming purposes, this oil is also known for reducing high blood pressure, stimulating hair growth, fighting intestinal problems, reducing nausea, soothing headaches, and reducing the effects of certain skin conditions.

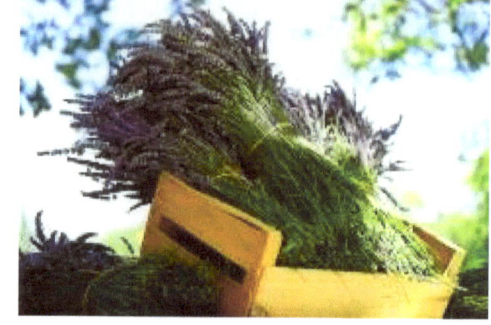

Lemon

It may not surprise you that lemon oil is one of the most popular essential oils on the market, considering the clean smell this fruit is known for.

This essential oil aids in digestion, improves concentration, and eases the symptoms of arthritis and acne. On top of that, it is also a natural immunity booster.

If you want to feel more energized throughout the day, you can simply add a few drops of lemon oil to your diffuser or vaporizer. If you want to boost your immune system, then you should include a few drops in your bathwater. Note that it's not that wise to use lemon oil in the sun.

Sandalwood

Due to its particularly woody fragrance, it's incredibly easy to recognize the smell of sandalwood. This is one of the more expensive essential oils because it is extracted only when a tree reaches maturity. However, if you can afford it, then you should definitely purchase it, as it offers numerous health benefits.

Sandalwood is best known for alleviating chest pain. It can also be used to relieve tension. It's worth noting that sandalwood also has anti-inflammatory properties and that it hydrates the skin.

Jasmine

Considering how beautiful jasmine smells, it comes as no surprise that this essential oil is best known for its relaxing properties. It isn't easy to make jasmine oil, which is the main reason why it's one of the most expensive oils available.

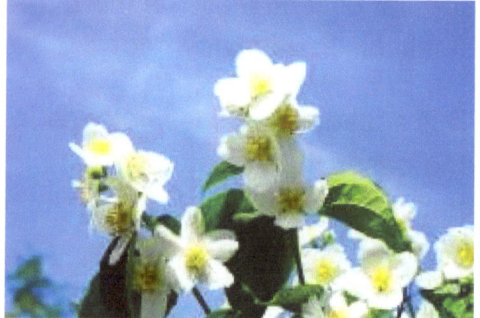

Jasmine is used for everything from a home air freshener to helping ease mild depression. It can also be used to help with addiction issues and respiratory problems. Pregnant women should avoid using this essential oil.

Rosemary

If you're feeling stressed out and you can't seem to focus properly, then you should add a few drops of rosemary oil to your bathwater or diffuser in order to relax. This essential oil can enhance memory and improve overall brain performance. You can also use rosemary oil to soothe cramping muscles, migraines, and headaches. If you're suffering from certain skin issues, you can benefit from using this essential oil.

Rosemary oil is noted for being one of the strongest essential oils, which is why pregnant women, as well as individuals with high blood pressure or epilepsy should avoid using it.

Peppermint

Whenever you feel that you're starting to lose focus, know that just a whiff of peppermint can get you back on track. There's a good reason why most chewing gum have a peppermint flavor. Once you smell this essential oil, you will instantly be refreshed.

It is mostly used to enhance mental alertness, although it can also combat redness and irritation, and even aid in digestion. Be cautious when applying peppermint oil; you should keep it away from your eyes!

Chamomile

Drinking a cup of chamomile tea during a cold winter's day is always relaxing. However, if you want to truly take some time to unwind, then you need to start using chamomile essential oil. This essential oil is used as an antidepressant, 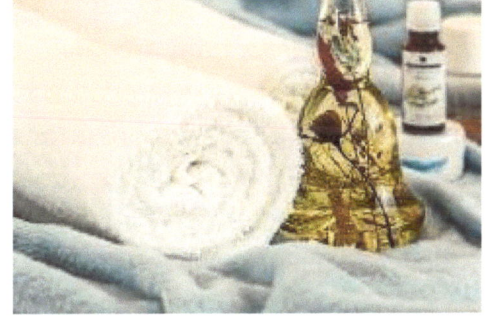 antiseptic, antibiotic, and mood lifter.

It can be used in a diffuser, steam therapy or a few drops in a bath, on a pillow or a handkerchief placed in a purse or pocket. You can blend it with massage oils or mix it with certain creams and lotions. You shouldn't use chamomile oil if you're allergic to ragweed or in the first trimester of pregnancy, ask your doctor.

Cedarwood

Cedarwood is an essential oil made from the Juniperus Virginiana tree that's been around since the time of ancient Egyptians. In fact, this is believed to be one of the first essential oils ever extracted. You can mix Cedarwood oil with facial creams or massage oil, but you can also add a few drops to your diffuser or vaporizer.

Cedarwood is best known for helping alleviate anxiety and stress. However, it can also aid respiratory problems and ease urinary tract infections. Note that this oil is a skin irritant and so must be diluted with a carrier oil, like almond, jojoba or avocado oil.

Marjoram

If you're suffering from anxiety problems or dealing with hyperactivity issues, then you should add a few drops of marjoram oil to your vaporizer or diffuser. On top of reducing anxiety, this essential oil also helps combat depression and fatigue. Not to mention that it alleviates circulatory and respiratory issues as well.

How to Use and Apply Essential Oils

There are numerous methods of application when it comes to essential oils. Here are some of the most popular ones:

Mixing Essential Oils With Massage Oil: Massages are always relaxing and offer you numerous health benefits by helping you reduce stress. However, when you mix essential oils with massage oil, you will experience even more benefits. Massages with essential oils will help enhance your immune system, relax your nervous system, treat headaches and migraines, and offer pain relief.

Steam Inhalation: Steam inhalation is a really simple way to use aromatherapy. You place 3 to 7 drops of essential oil into boiling water, cover your head with a towel, close your eyes, and breathe through the nose. Steam inhalation will help enhance respiratory function.

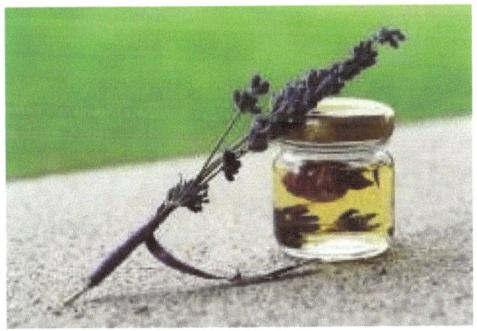

Inhalation Methods: There are different ways to inhale essential oils. You can inhale directly from your palm, from the bottle, place a few drops on your pillow and inhale deeply before you fall asleep. You can also place a few drops on a tissue or handkerchief and inhale, take it with you in your purse or pocket. Inhalation will not only help improve respiratory function, but it will also help you relax and improve your mood.

Diffuser Inhalation: Diffusers are special machines that diffuse essential oils into the air for inhalation. There are different models available and each uses a specific delivery method. Using diffusers will help improve your energy levels, increase alertness, improve your mood, boost sleep quality, and fill your home, office, or car with healing air-freshening aromas.

Add To Showers: Plug your drain, and add a few drops of oil to the floor of your shower and create a therapeutic steam that will envelop your whole body.

Facial Creams And Lotions: If you want to rejuvenate your skin, you can simply buy unscented body lotions and facial creams and mix them with essential oils. Mixing them together will improve your skin tone, slow down the aging of the skin, reduce the visibility of scars, increase local circulation, and encourage hydration of the skin.

Baths: Adding 5 to 12 drops of essential oils into your bath can provide you with a number of health benefits. Most importantly, it will help reduce stress and anxiety, while also alleviating you of muscular tension and pain. Other health benefits of adding essential oils to your bath include increased local circulation, detoxification, and improved skin health.

Different Types of Aromatherapy Diffusers

Nebulizing Diffusers

Nebulizing diffusers put out large quantities of essential oil
particles into the air.
Usually in this model, a
bottle of oil is attached to
the unit and so unfiltered
and undiluted oil streams
into the air. Because this
type of diffusion allows
whole oil to diffuse into

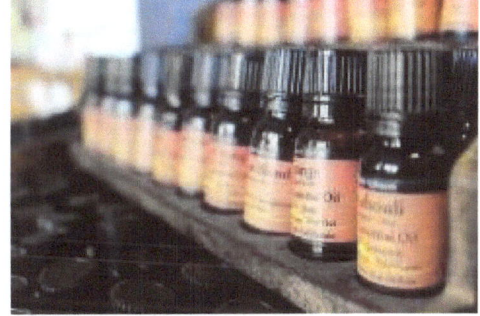

the air, it is the best method of getting therapeutic use out of
essential oils.

If you're doing aromatherapy for therapeutic reasons, then
you should probably go with this type of diffusion because it
uses no water, no filtration and therefore puts the highest
amount of essential oils into the air.

Although these kinds of diffusers are generally considered
the best choice, they do have a somewhat big downside.
Namely, since they are so powerful and do a good job of
saturating the air with essential oils, they are sometimes a bit
on the noisy side and some models use up oil at a high rate.
Nevertheless, this shouldn't be viewed as a problem.
Nebulizers typically have built-in timers so the unit only runs
for a set of amount of minutes per hour, which helps save oil
without sacrificing its therapeutic value.

Ultrasonic or Humidifying Diffusers

Ultrasonic diffusers come with a tank that requires water and essential oil added to this tank. While the scent is still evident, the use of water actually means that much less of therapeutic oil actually reaches the air, and your nose and body. Typically, these models are less expensive than nebulizing diffusers.

Evaporative Diffusers

Evaporative diffusers use a filter pad where drops of oil are placed and a built-in fan blows onto the pad causing the oil to evaporate and blow into the air.

Even though evaporative diffusers are generally considered to be a good and somewhat quiet way to get essential oils into the air in your home, they do have a downside. Namely, when an essential oil begins to evaporate, the lighter components of it will evaporate first, only to be followed by the heavier components later. Therefore, basically, the air in your home will be filled with lighter components in the beginning and with heavier components later on. This means that you may actually lose some of the therapeutic properties the whole oil possesses.

These models typically require the use of more oil to get a similar effect as compared to nebulizing diffusers and also cost more in maintenance since the filters need to be replaced.

Heat Diffusers

These models use heat instead of air to diffuse oils into the air. Heat diffusers are popular because they are very economical and they're completely silent when working.

However, they share the same downside as evaporative diffusers, namely lighter components of essential oils evaporate before the heavier ones. Nevertheless, if the noise a diffuser makes is something that bothers you, and you want a completely silent and very economical unit, then these models are with looking into.

Key Tips for Essential Oils

We already discussed some of the essential oils, their healing properties and how to use them. Here are a few other key tips to using essential oils.

Blending Essential Oils

Blending oils is a great way to gain various therapeutic benefits from a single oil. You can make your own blends, or buy ready-made blends that target specific needs.

Use High Quality Oils

Use only 100% pure therapeutic grade essential oils, from reputable brands. Therapeutic grade oils are your best option, unlike lower quality products that use fillers to reduce cost, but also diminish the therapeutic value that is in pure oils. As far as quality goes, due diligence and careful research pays off.

Precautions

Essential oils come in many flavors and are incredibly strong substances, so they must be mixed with a carrier oil (in most cases coconut, almond, or jojoba oil) before they are applied to the skin to avoid irritation.

The safety of ingesting essential oils depends on the flavor of oil, again due diligence and careful research pays off in this case, so always check before using any oil internally.

The same goes if you are pregnant, ask your doctor before using essential oils. Cinnamon, rosemary, clove, and clary sage, should be avoided by pregnant women as they can cause contractions.

10 Dangerous Oils to Avoid

There are oils that are not appropriate for consumption or for topical use and can be dangerous in these instances because they can be poisonous and cause skin irritations:

- Bitter Almond
- Calamus
- Yellow Camphor
- Savin
- Southernwood
- Tansy
- Mugwort
- Mustard
- Rue
- Horseradish

Avoid using these oils!

101 Ways to Use Essential Oils

Household Uses

1. Eliminate Shower Scum – Add 4 drops of eucalyptus essential oil, 4 drops of tea tree oil and 1/2 cup of baking soda to warm water in a spray bottle. Spray around your shower to eliminate shower scum.

2. Purify Air – Cinnamon essential oil contains anti-microbial properties making it a great choice to use in a diffuser to clean the air in your home.

3. Outdoor Furniture Scrub – In a spray bottle, combine 20 drops of juniper berry, 20 drops of lemon essential oil, and 20 drops of pine essential oil. Mix with 2 tablespoons of white vinegar and top off with water. Shake well and spray liberally onto patio furniture.

4. Eliminate Lingering Cooking Odors – Place a pan of water on the stove, cook to a simmer and then add 4 to 5 drops of citrus, lemongrass or clove essential oil to the water.

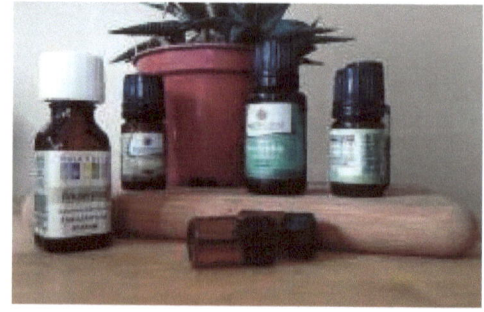

5. Window Wash – Combine twelve drops of lemon essential oil with one ounce of white vinegar, and one ounce of water. Use in a spray bottle to clean windows and mirrors.

6. All Purpose Cleaner – Lemongrass and tea tree oil are natural disinfectants. Make your own natural cleaning solution by adding a few drops of these oils to warm water, works great for kitchen and bathroom counters.

7. Clean Sports Gear – Use 3 drops of tea tree oil and 2 drops of lemon essential oil mixed with one quart of warm water and 5 tablespoons of baking soda to wash foul smelling sports gear.

8. Better Smelling Laundry – Add 15 to 20 drops of your preferred essential oil into each load for fresh smelling laundry.

9. Refresh Your Vacuum Cleaner – Put 5 to 10 drops of your favorite essential oil into your vacuum's bag or dust container.

10. Bathtub Scrub – Combine 5 drops of bergamot oil or lime oil with one-half of a cup of baking soda and one-half cup of vinegar. Use this mixture to scrub your bathroom sink, toilet, or bathtub.

11. Wash Produce – Lemon oil is an antiseptic so you use 2 drops per large bowl of warm water to wash insecticide and dirt off your produce.

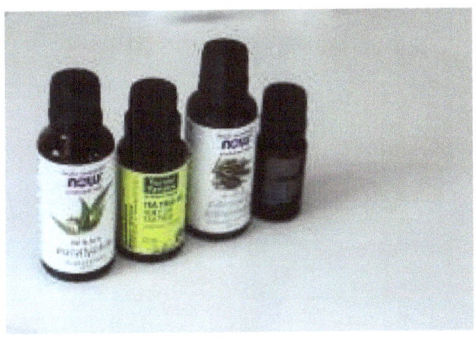

12. Freshen The Trash Can – Place 4 drops of lemon essential oil and 5 drops of tea tree oil onto a cotton ball.

13. Place the cotton ball at the bottom of the trashcan to help eliminate odors and detoxify.

14. Grout Scrub – Combine ten drops of eucalyptus oil with one part castile soap, one part water, and four parts baking soda. Use to clean grout.

15. Neutralize Pet Odor – Use 10 to 20 drops of either geranium, lavender, or lemon oil with apple cider vinegar. Shake well and spray around the room that you wish to eliminate pet odor.

16. Fridge Purifier – To keep your fridge smelling clean after you wash it, add a few drops of lime or grapefruit oil to warm water and wipe all parts of fridge. Do this regularly to enjoy the fresh smell all the time.

17. Cleaner Dishes – Place a few drops of lemon essential oil in your dishwasher before running to ensure a spot-free rinse.

18. Eliminate Mold – Place tea tree oil in your diffuser to kill mold and other pathogens in the air. You can also mix tea tree oil with water and spray on any mold spots around your home to kill the spores.

19. Remove Mites From Bedding – Place a few drops of eucalyptus essential oil to your washing machine when you are washing your bedding.

20. Remove Cigarette Smoke Odor – Place four drops each of rosemary essential oil, tea tree oil, and eucalyptus essential oil to a spray bottle filled with water and spray around the house.

21. Air-Freshener – Add your favorite oils to an aromatherapy diffuser to freshen the air at your home and also enjoy the benefits of the therapeutic value of aromatherapy.

22. Mosquito Repellent – Add 1 drop of citronella oil, 1 drop of lemongrass oil and 1 drop of eucalyptus oil to 1 tablespoon of coconut oil and apply to skin.

23. Homemade Sunscreen – Combine coconut oil, Shea butter, helichrysum oil, zinc oxide and lavender oil, and store in a squeeze bottle.

24. Deter Flying Insects – Place two cups of potpourri in a decorative bowl. Place ten to fifteen drops of citronella essential oil in the potpourri and place in an area you want to deter flying insects.

25. Mouse Repellent – Mix two tablespoons of peppermint essential oil with one cup of water in a spray bottle. Spritz the mixture anywhere you have seen mouse droppings and especially behind appliances.

26. Deodorize Upholstery – Place a few drops of your choice of essential oil into one cup of baking soda. Sprinkle onto your upholstery and let set for fifteen minutes. Vacuum off.

27. Furniture Dusting Spray – Place one and three quarters of a cup of filtered water into a spray bottle. Add two teaspoons of olive oil, one-half of a teaspoon of lemon essential oil and one quarter of a cup of vinegar. Mix well and use to remove dust from furniture.

28. Flavored Water – Put two to three drops of lemon essential oil to your drinking water for a delicious citrus flavor.

29. Natural Dryer Sheets – Mix one cup of pure distilled vinegar with 15 drops of lavender or rose essential oil. Place cloth scraps into the mixture until they are moistened but not soaked. Add one cloth per dryer load.

Health And Wellness

30. Improve Sleep – Place a few drops of lavender essential oil on your pillow to help you fall asleep and sleep better throughout the night. Lavender is known for helping to alleviate insomnia.

31. Relieve Stress and Tension – Use lavender and chamomile oils in a diffuser, or place a few drops on a tissue and inhale regularly. Adding a few drops to a hot bath is wonderful for alleviating stress, tension and related body aches.

32. Massage Oil – Add a few drops of Cedarwood essential oil to an unscented lotion or massage oil and use for a relaxing massage.

33. Detox Bath – Adding lavender essential oil, Epsom salts, and sea salts to a warm bath will cleanse and rejuvenate the body.

34. Headaches – For migraines and headaches, mix rosemary, eucalyptus, peppermint, and/or sandalwood oils with a carrier oil, like Jojoba and rub into your temples or scalp.

35. Improve Depression – Adding rose essential oils to a bath, inhalations, and diffusers will boost mood and relieve depression.

36. Calm Children – Placing a couple drops of lavender or chamomile essential oils on stuffed animals can help to soothe and calm an upset child.

37. Lighten The Mood – Placing lavender, rose, ylang-ylang, chamomile, or orange essential oil in a diffuser brightens mood and improves positive energy in any room.

38. Stay Alert – To help you stay alert, inhale the scent of lavender, sage, frankincense, lemon, peppermint, lemongrass, and basil essential oils in any combination.

39. Foot Soak – To help ease sore and tired feet, place your feet in warm water that contains peppermint essential oil and Epsom salts.

40. Bolster Your Immune System – Rubbing oregano essential oil to the bottoms of your feet can help to bolster your immune system.

41. Relax Tired Muscles – A warm bath with eucalyptus, sage, and basil essential oils will help to relax your tired muscles.

42. Improve Circulation – Adding 8 to 10 drops of grapefruit essential oils to a warm bath will help to improve your circulation.

43. Lose Weight – To aid in weight loss, inhale peppermint, and cinnamon essential oils to reduce your appetite and balance your blood sugars.

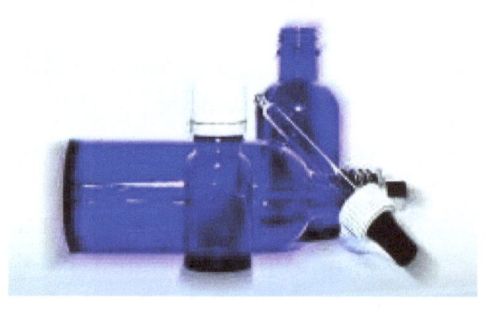

44. Reduce Anxiety – Diffusing lavender essential oil around your house can help to combat feelings of stress and tension.

45. Control Anger – Diffuse jasmine, patchouli, bergamot, or rose essential oils around your home to help with anger management.

46. Increase Confidence – To help increase your confidence, diffuse cypress, grapefruit, or rosemary essential oils around your home.

47. Control Fear – To help with feelings of fear, diffuse frankincense, neroli, or sandalwood essential oils.

48. Cope With Grief – To help with the grieving process, diffuse Helichrysum, neroli, or vetiver essential oils. You can also include these oils in a warm bath to aid relaxation as you grieve.

49. Increase Memory And Concentration – To help aid memory and concentration while you are studying, diffuse black pepper, hyssop, or peppermint essential oils.

Beauty And Healthcare

50. Body Butter – Make a body butter by combining Shea butter, cocoa butter, coconut oil, and thirty drops of your choice of essential oils. This combination will leave your skin moisturized for days.

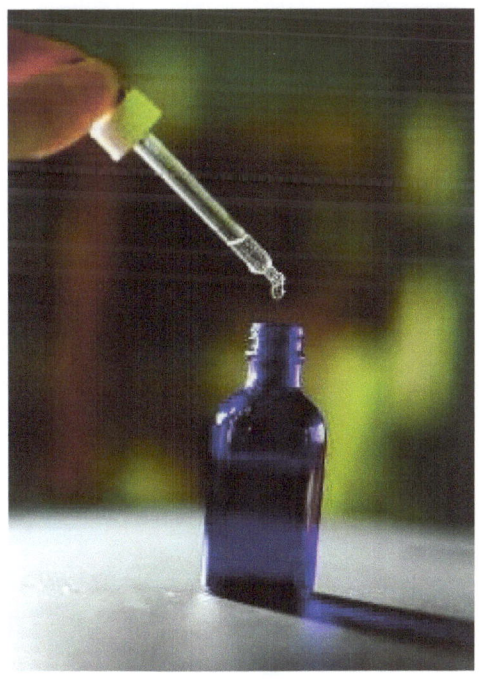

51. Lip Balm – A combination of coconut oil, beeswax, and lavender essential oil will help to heal chapped and dry lips.

52. ace Toner – For a natural face toner, combine eight ounces of water with two drops each of lavender, geranium, and frankincense essential oils. Apply daily.

53. Body Mist – Combine about ten drops of your choice of essential oils to fifty milliliters of water in a small spray bottle. Mix well before using.

54. Fight Acne – Combine aloe vera gel with a few drops of tea tree essential oil and apply to acne-prone areas twice a day.

55. Hair Growth Oil – Placing one to two drops of carrot essential oil to your hairbrush daily before brushing will help promote healthy hair growth.

56. Anti-Aging – Mix one to two drops of either almond, rosemary or lavender essential oils to your night cream and apply daily.

57. Perfume – Use one to two drops of jasmine, lavender, or vanilla essential oils on your wrist for a natural perfume. Cypress and clove essential oils are good options for men.

58. Shampoo – Combine lavender and rosemary essential oils to coconut milk and aloe vera gel to make a homemade shampoo that will last for two to four week. Use as a regular shampoo.

59. Freshen Breath – A single drop of peppermint essential oil works as a natural way to freshen your breath.

60. Deodorant – Coconut oil combined with beeswax and your choice of essential oil can be used as a natural deodorant.

61. Wrinkle Reducer – Add 4 to 6 drops each of geranium, sandalwood, lavender and frankincense essential oils to an unscented facial cream. Apply to face daily, avoiding the eyes.

62. Prevent Hair Loss – Combining your choice of burdock root, ginger, lavender, rosemary, thyme or yarrow essential oils can be mixed with a carrier oil and applied to your hair to reduce thinning.

63. Sugar Scrub – Make a homemade sugar scrub, which is economical and effective. Simply add 4 drops of your favorite essential oils and 4 drops of vitamin E or jojoba oil to ½ a cup of sugar and mix together. Use as an exfoliant for the face and body to scrub away dead skin cells.

64. Thicken Hair – Adding a few drops of rosemary to your favorite shampoo with help to naturally add volume to your hair and thicken it.

65. Relieve Dry Scalp – Place a few drops of lavender, Cedarwood or basil essential oils to your shampoo to moisturize your scalp and reduce itching.

66. Treat Dandruff – Add 5 drops of rosemary and lavender essential oils to 3 tablespoons of jojoba oil. Blend well, and massage into the scalp, let sit for 10 minutes, then shampoo as usual. Repeat weekly.

67. Reduce Age Spots – Massage frankincense oil directly on sunspots and age spots three times a day to lighten them.

68. Reduce Stretch Marks – Combine 5 drops each of myrrh, grapefruit, and frankincense essential oils into coconut oil and apply to stretch marks daily to reduce their appearance.

69. Hair Detangling Spray – In a spray bottle, combine eight ounces of distilled water, one teaspoon of aloe vera gel, two drops of glycerin, and five drops each of lavender and rosemary essential oils. Spray onto hair as needed.

70. Baby Shampoo – Combine two ounces of Castile baby soap, one-teaspoon jojoba oil, and 10 drops of the essential oil of your choice. Use as a gentle option to wash baby's hair and skin.

71. Deep Hair Conditioner – Combine 8 drops of an essential oil of your choice, lavender has a great scent, with three tablespoons of coconut oil and one tablespoon of olive oil. Allow to sit on your hair for fifteen minutes. Rinse, shampoo, and style as desired.

72. Toothpaste – Make a homemade toothpaste with a mixture of sea salt, coconut oil, baking soda, and peppermint essential oil.

73. Goodbye Cellulite – To help reduce the appearance of cellulite, combine 7 drops of grapefruit essential oil with 2 tablespoons of coconut oil, and massage into affected areas.

74. Eczema Relief – A mixture of lavender oil and Shea butter is an effective treatment for eczema, psoriasis, and red dry skin.

75. Tinted Lip Balm – Combine 25 drops of your favorite essential oil with three tablespoons of coconut oil, two tablespoons of beeswax, one tablespoon each of jojoba oil and beetroot powder and you will have a naturally tinted lip balm.

76. Serum For Firmer Skin – Combine one and a half tablespoons of aloe vera gel, one teaspoon of strong coffee, two drops of cypress essential oil and one teaspoon of witch hazel. Apply this treatment to your face every morning.

77. Hand Soap – Combine a few drops of your favorite essential oil with five parts water and one part liquid castile soap and place in a foaming hand dispenser.

78. Homemade Hand Sanitizer – Combine 6 drops of lavender and 25 drops of tea tree essential oils with 1 teaspoon of vitamin E oil and 8 ounces of aloe vera gel, it's fine to use gel directly from the plant.

79. Herbal Bath Salts – Add 20 to 30 drops of your favorite essential oils to one cup of Epsom salts and ½ cup of natural sea salt. Place in a glass container with a tight fitting lid. Add ½ cup to each warm bath.

Homemade Remedies

80. Homemade Vapor Rub – Combine 1/2 a cup of coconut oil with about ten drops of eucalyptus oil and fifteen drops of peppermint essential oil.

    Apply to the chest as needed.

81. Get Rid Of Head Lice – Mix 3 drops each of lavender, thyme, and eucalyptus essential oils with a carrier oil, like jojoba or avocado oil and message into the scalp. Put on a shower cap and let sit for thirty minutes. Shampoo out, and comb out nits and bugs from hair with a fine toothcomb.

82. Cure Nausea – To ease nausea, breath in peppermint oil through your nose. You can also apply peppermint oil to your neck and upper chest to alleviate nausea.

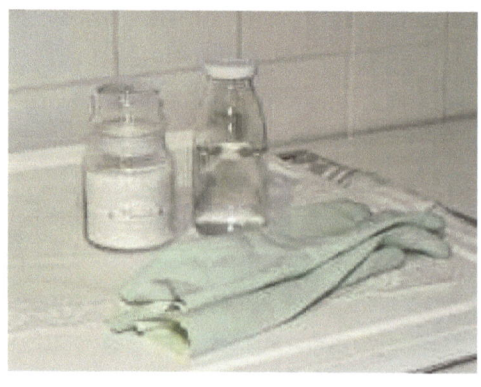

83. Relieve Menstrual Cramps – Combine 2 drops each of clary sage, basil, or rosemary essential oil with ½ cup of jojoba or avocado carrier oil. Massage the oil mixture into your abdomen, then cover with a towel soaked in warm water and let sit for 10 minutes. Repeat as needed throughout the day.

84. Insomnia – Diffuse chamomile or lavender oil in your bedroom, add a few drops to a hot pre-sleep bath, or place a few drops on your pillow.

85. Open Airways – Inhale the vapor of lavender and eucalyptus oils mixed with hot water to open the airways when you have congestion, a cold, or flu or really, anytime you wish to open airway passages and breathe better.

86. Disinfect Cuts – Dilute lavender or tea tree essential oils one to one in a carrier oil and use to disinfect cuts and scrapes.

87. Reduce Fever – Add equal parts of frankincense, peppermint, and sage to a warm bath. As an alternative, mix the same oils into lukewarm water and sponge onto feverish skin to reduce the fever.

88. Loosen Stiff Joints – Gently massage one teaspoon of a carrier oil mixed with a couple of drops of vetiver essential oil into stiff joints to encourage movement.

89. Cough Reducer – Mix three drops of eucalyptus and two drops of rosemary essential oil with one teaspoon of a carrier oil. Massage the mixture over the chest, back, throat and sinus area to relieve a cough.

90. Help Health Broken Bones – Apply fir and cypress essential oils to the area of a broken bone to support healing.

91. Heal Burns – Combine lavender essential oil and aloe vera to treat minor burns. Apply liberally to burned area.

92. Reduce Bug Bite Itch – Apply lavender essential oil to bug bites to help reduce the itch.

93. Boost Digestive Health - Clove oil taken with meals helps reduce digestive discomfort as it contains 95% eugenol that fights various fungal over growths that can disrupt healthy digestive function. It also helps relax the smooth muscle lining of the digestive tract to prevent gas, bloating, nausea and diarrhea, bloating, and gas. Clove oil is antiviral, antifungal, and antibacterial so it can help kill pathogens that play a key role in digestive problems.

94. Treat Bruises – Add five drops each of lavender and frankincense to four ounces of hot water and soak a cloth in the mixture. Apply the cloth to the bruised area.

95. Teeth Grinding – Massage 1 to 3 drops of lavender oil to the bottom of the feet and behind the ears before bed to reduce teeth grinding in your sleep.

96. Hangovers – To alleviate the symptoms of a hangover, take a warm bath with 5 drops each of Cedarwood, lavender, rosemary, juniper berry, and lemon essential oils.

97. Treat Cold Sores – Lavender is antibacterial, antiviral, and antifungal as well as a natural pain reliever and an anti-itch remedy. Apply one drop to a cold sore as soon as you notice it forming to help heal the cold sore. Apply as needed.

98. Treat Ear Aches – Add 1 drop of lavender and chamomile essential oils to warmed olive oil and blend well, drop some of the mixture to a cotton ball and place on the outer ear canal.

    Add the rest of the mixture to another cotton ball and rub the external area behind the ear.

99. Treat Tendonitis – To help ease the pain from tendonitis, massage in a mixture of 3 tablespoons of a carrier oil, 5 drops of peppermint oil, 4 drops each of rosemary and eucalyptus oils, 8 drops of chamomile oil, and 3 drops of lavender oil.

100. Relieve Arthritis Pain – Add 2 drops of rosemary oil, 1 drop of lavender oil and 2 drops of chamomile oil to 1 to 2 tablespoons of Jojoba oil or any one of your favorite carrier oils. Massage the oil onto the area that hurts, and then place a warm towel over the area for 10 minutes.

101. Treat Neuralgia – First, apply an ice pack to numb the pain. Then massage the following mixture into the affected area: two drops of rosemary oil, one drop each of peppermint, chamomile, and lavender oils and one teaspoon of a carrier oil.

102. Allergy Relief – Rub one drop each of frankincense and lavender on your palms and inhale deeply. This will relieve itchy eyes and throat.

Final Thoughts

People have been using essential oils for more than 6,000 years, and aromatherapy is only getting more popular, so it's safe to say that it's a proven way to increase quality of life, and to promote healing and general wellness.

Some of the most notable health benefits you can experience by using essential oils include improved sleep quality, positive mood, happiness, improved memory, 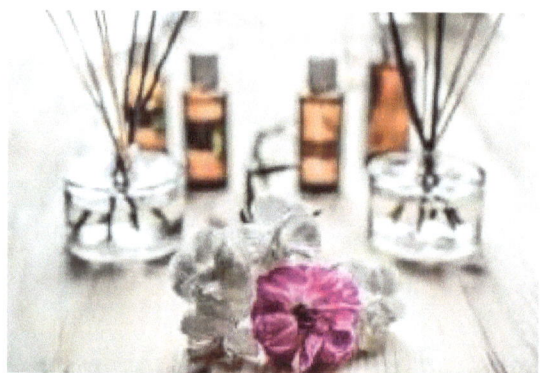 pain relief, improved skin health, increased energy levels and a general feeling of wellness and wellbeing.

Even if you're only looking for a way to relax after a stressful day, then aromatherapy will certainly do the trick!

Get started today!

Other Relevant Books by This Author

If you would like to read more about Senior Health and Fitness, here is a list of the CreateSpace links, titles and descriptions:

https://www.createspace.com/5714434

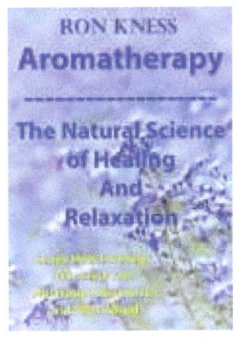 **Aromatherapy - The Science of Healing and Relaxation: Learn How Essential Oils Elicit The Relaxation Response And Alter Mood**

In my book, we reveal the natural holistic methods you can use to heal the body from certain medical issues and to relive stress through relaxation. In particular we talk about:

• Aromatherapy - what it is and how it works
• Essential Oils – how the effects of certain aromas differs from others
• Recipes – how to make your own essential oil combinations

https://www.createspace.com/6419369

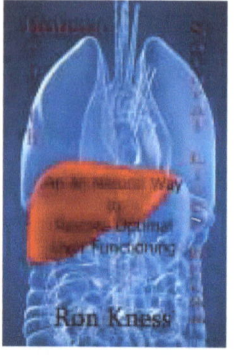

Natural Liver Detox: An All-Natural Way to Restore Optimal Liver Functioning

We live in a world that is chocked-full of toxins be it in the air we breathe, our food, our water… so much so that their entrance into our bodies has become unavoidable.

Exposure to these toxins requires that all of the organs in your body work in synergy to maintain homeostasis - meaning everything needs to be in a certain balance in order to function optimally. If the function of one organ or system goes awry, the others will also be affected.

Your liver and kidneys play a vital role of filtering toxins out of your body, but your liver has an additional function of breaking down the present toxins in order to expel them from your body.

This enzymatic process occurs in two phases – breaking down the toxins and bonding these broken parts to other molecules that destroy the toxic substances and expel them from your body through sweat, urine and fecal matter.

When the liver becomes overburdened or overworked due to chronic exposure to toxins via the environment, diet, smoking, alcohol use, lack of sleep or poor stress management, it can slow down and cause a back-up of toxins in your system. This can impact many other systems and organs in your body resulting in various symptoms.

In this book we show you the signs that your liver may be struggling, how to set up a detox plan and the foods to eat to help keep it operating at optimal efficiency.

https://www.createspace.com/6433160

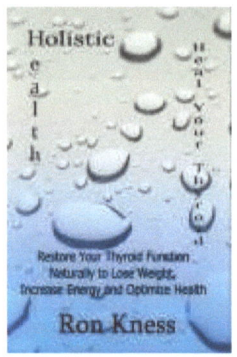

Heal Your Thyroid: Restore Your Thyroid Function Naturally to Lose Weight, Increase Energy and Optimize Health

The thyroid is a gland that is responsible for regulating many of your bodily functions and if it isn't functioning properly, you will experience a variety of symptoms that can impact your life in unfavorable ways.

The problem is that diagnosing a thyroid disorder can be difficult because the symptoms can be vague and attributed to many different things. Because of this, millions of people wake up every day with thyroid issues without even knowing it:

- Do you constantly feel so fatigued that you barely have the energy to brush your teeth?

- Do you find that there is more hair than usual ending up in your brush or shower drain?

- Are you gaining weight or just not losing no matter how much you try to adapt a healthy lifestyle?

- Do you often feel cold or have sensitivity to cold temperatures?

- Do you have constant brain fog or memory issues?

- Do you have dry eyes?

Well most of us experience these things at various times and because we simply assume that age is catching up with us or that we are not exercising as frequently as we should or that we are not getting enough sleep…we just chalk them up to something we have to live with and don't pursue any medical follow-up.

Many times it is an under-performing thyroid that is causing problems. With the proper nutrition, exercise and some lifestyle changes, you can heal your thyroid. They are all things you should be doing anyway, so what do you have to lose?

https://www.createspace.com/6528679

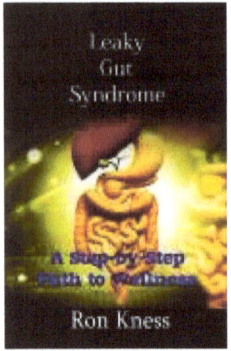

Leaky Gut Syndrome - Could This Be Why You Are Sick?: A Step-by-Step Path to Wellness

Leaky gut is just now starting to come onto the radar for doctors as more and more people are developing gastrointestinal and other disorders with no known cause. If you have frequent unexplained sickness, you could have leaky gut syndrome.

What it means is things are getting through the wall of the small intestine that aren't supposed to get through.

One of the big jobs of your small intestine is to finish the digestive process by continuing to break down the food you have eaten into smaller and smaller particles. And then, it absorbs the nutrients from that food through your intestinal wall and into your bloodstream where the nutrients can be absorbed by cells and converted into energy.

And it has another big job, too. It's supposed to keep harmful stuff inside the tube, where it can't cause too much trouble for your immune system. Things like bad germs, toxins, and food particles that are still too big for your body to use.

But sometimes, the lining of the small intestine gets damaged or the communication signals get confused resulting in things get through that shouldn't. And that can turn into even bigger problems in the form of infection or autoimmune disorders.

But in this guide, you will learn about what the leaky gut syndrome is, its potential causes, and proposed treatments that might be able to not only relieve your symptoms, but make leaky gut a thing of the past.

About the Author

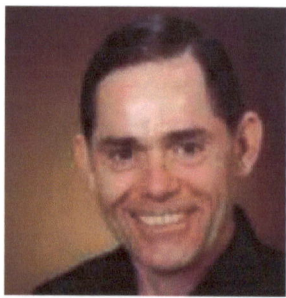

I grew up in Central Minnesota, where my parents owned and operated a fishing resort. Once out of high school I tried a couple of semesters of college, only to quit halfway through the Spring term; I decided at that time that college wasn't for me.

Then I decided to follow my father's previous occupation as an auto mechanic. I graduated from a two-year of vocational training course and worked as a mechanic for five years. While in vocational training, I decided to join the National Guard where I eventually ended up working full-time for 32 years.

So how does all of this relate to writing? In one of my leadership schools, the instructor, who was an English teacher at a juvenile detention center, presented writing to me in a whole new way - a way that started to develop my interest in working with words.

I eventually went back to college on the GI Bill while I was working and earned my Bachelor's degree in Business Administration. Taking a class or two per semester at night and on weekends took me seven years to complete my degree.

Fast forward about 40 years and I now have published over 75 books on Amazon for Kindle, CreateSpace and other publishing platforms.

Besides my own writing, I also ghostwrite ebooks, reports, articles, blogs and do Kindle conversions for clients on a variety of topics.

Today my wife and I are retired from our careers and live in Gold Canyon, AZ. I now write as a retirement business where you'll find me happily sitting in my office typing away on my laptop as I work on my next book or ghostwriting project . . . that is if we are not traveling on a cruise ship - our new-found mode of travel.

www.ingramcontent.com/pod-product-compliance
Lightning Source LLC
Chambersburg PA
CBHW050829290526
45792CB00001B/318

* 9 7 8 1 5 4 0 6 6 6 1 6 1 *